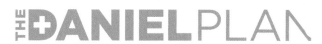

SERIES

FAITH

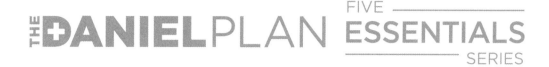

THE DANIEL PLAN

FIVE ESSENTIALS SERIES

FAITH

Essential One

NURTURING YOUR SOUL

STUDY GUIDE · FOUR SESSIONS

featuring

GARY THOMAS
& DEE EASTMAN

with KAREN LEE-THORP

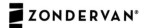

ZONDERVAN®

ZONDERVAN

Faith Study Guide
Copyright © 2015 by The Daniel Plan

This title is also available as a Zondervan ebook. Visit www.zondervan.com/ebooks.

Requests for information should be addressed to:
Zondervan, 3900 *Sparks Dr. SE*, Grand Rapids, Michigan 49546

ISBN 978-0-310-81995-0

Cover photography: iStockphoto
Interior photography: Robert Ortiz, Kent Cameron, Don Haynes, Robert Hawkins, Shelly Antol, Matt Armendariz, the PICS Ministry at Saddleback Church, iStockphoto
Interior design: Kait Lamphere

First Printing May 2015 / Printed in the United States of America

Contents

Welcome Letter

I am so glad you have joined us for this Daniel Plan study. I am excited for your journey, as I have seen firsthand that change is within reach as you embrace the Daniel Plan lifestyle. This groundbreaking program will equip you with practical tools to bring health into every area of your life. It has been transformative for thousands of people around the world and can be for you as well.

I speak from experience. I've not only witnessed endless stories of life change but have personally benefited from these Daniel Plan Essentials for many years now. Working full-time with five grown children, including identical triplet girls, I understand what it is like to juggle many priorities and have my health impacted. The key elements of The Daniel Plan have been completely restorative in my life as I have integrated them one step at a time.

As you go through this four-week study, the perfect complement to maximize your success is reading *The Daniel Plan: 40 Days to a Healthier Life*. The book includes a 40-day food and fitness guide, complete with a meal plan, recipes, shopping lists, and exercises that will energize your efforts. It will complement any of The Daniel Plan studies you dive into. There are also numerous articles and free resources on our website (www.danielplan.com), along with a weekly newsletter filled with tools and inspiration to keep you flourishing.

Congratulations on taking the next step to gaining vitality in your life. My prayer is that you will be inspired and fully equipped to continue your journey, and that you will experience a whole new level of wellness in the process. I pray that you will feel God's presence and will be reenergized to follow all he has planned for you.

For His Glory,

Dee Eastman

Dee Eastman
Founding Director, The Daniel Plan

How to Use This Guide

There are five video studies in The Daniel Plan series, one for each of the five Essentials (Faith, Food, Fitness, Focus, and Friends). Each study is four sessions long. The studies may be done in any order. If your group is new, consider starting with the six-week *The Daniel Plan Study Guide* and companion DVD, which offers an overview of all five Essentials.

GROUP SIZE

Each Daniel Plan video study is designed to be experienced in a group setting such as a Bible study, Sunday school class, or any small group gathering. To ensure that everyone has enough time to participate in discussions, it is recommended that large groups break into smaller groups of four to six people each.

MATERIALS NEEDED

Each participant should have his or her own study guide, which includes notes for video segments, directions for activities, discussion questions, and ideas for personal application between sessions. This curriculum is best used in conjunction with *The Daniel Plan: 40 Days to a Healthier Life*, which includes a complete 40-day food and fitness guide that complements this study.

TIMING

Each session is designed to be completed in 60 to 90 minutes, depending on your setting and the size of your group. Each video is approximately 20 minutes long.

OUTLINE OF EACH SESSION

Each group session will include the following:

» *Coming Together.* The foundation for spiritual growth is an intimate connection with God and his family. A few people who really know you and earn your trust provide a place to experience the life Jesus invites you to live. This opening portion of your meeting is an opportunity to transition from your busy life into your group time.

In Session 1 you'll find some icebreaker questions on the session topic, along with guidelines that state the values your group will live by so that everyone feels comfortable sharing. In Sessions 2 – 4 you'll have a chance to check in with other group members to report praise and progress toward your goals of healthy living. You'll also be able to share how you chose to put the previous session's insights into practice – and what the results were. There's no pressure for everyone to answer. This is time to get to know each other better and cheer each other on.

» *Learning Together.* This is the time when you will view the video teaching segment. This study guide provides notes on the key points of the video teaching along with space for you to write additional thoughts and questions.

» *Growing Together.* Here is where you will discuss the teaching you watched. The focus will be on how the teaching intersects with your real life.

» *What I Want to Remember.* You'll have a couple of minutes after your discussion to write down one or two key insights from the teaching and discussion that you want to remember.

» *Better Together.* The Daniel Plan is all about transforming the way you actually live. So before you close your meeting in prayer, you'll take some time to think about how you might apply what you've discussed. Under "Next Steps" you'll find a list of things you can do to put the session's insights into practice. Then the "Food Tip of the Week" offers a bonus video with a great recipe or food idea. It is on your DVD if you want to view it together with your group. It is also available online for you to view on your own during the week. Likewise, the "Fitness Move of the Week" is a bonus video with a simple exercise you can add to your fitness practices. It, too, is on your DVD and online.

Encourage each other to be specific about one or two things you plan to do each week as next steps. Consider asking someone in the group to be your buddy to hold each other accountable. Create an atmosphere of fun and positive reinforcement.

» *Praying Together.* The group session will close with time for a response to God in prayer, thanking him for what he's doing for you and asking for his help to live out what you have learned. Ideas for group prayer, as well as a written closing prayer, are provided. Feel free to use them or not. Consider having different group members lead the prayer time.

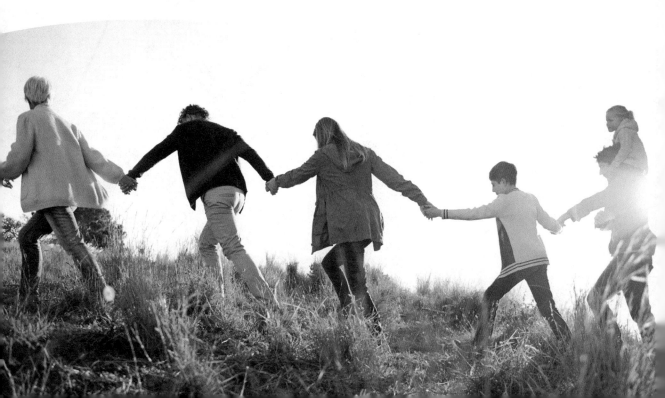

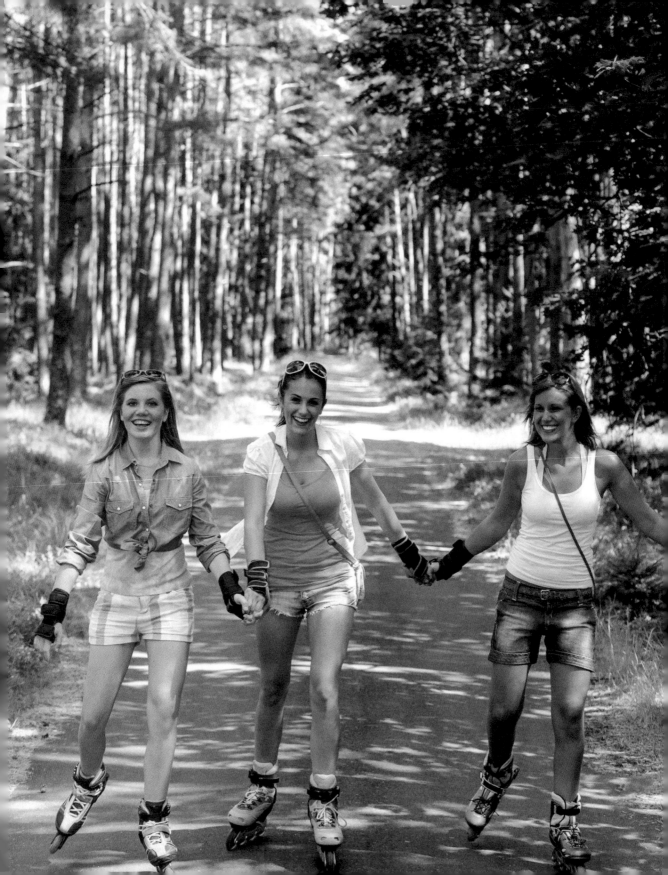

Every Body Matters

> "Do you not know that your bodies are temples of the Holy Spirit, who is in you, whom you have received from God?"
> 1 Corinthians 6:19

Did you know that God cares about our bodies, not just our souls? God made our bodies. He designed us to be embodied. He knit us together in our mothers' wombs (Psalm 139:13). And Jesus himself took on a human body: "The Word became flesh and made his dwelling among us" (John 1:14). He rose from the dead with a body (Luke 24:36–43) and ascended into heaven with his body (Luke 24:50–51). God loves our bodies.

In this study on Faith, we'll learn about spiritual health and its connection to physical health. We'll begin in this session by looking at God's calling for us to offer our bodies to him as living sacrifices.

COMING
TOGETHER

If this is your first time meeting together as a group, take a moment to introduce yourself.

Also, pass around a sheet of paper on which each person can write his or her name, address, phone number, and email address. Ask for a volunteer to type up the list and email it to everyone else this week.

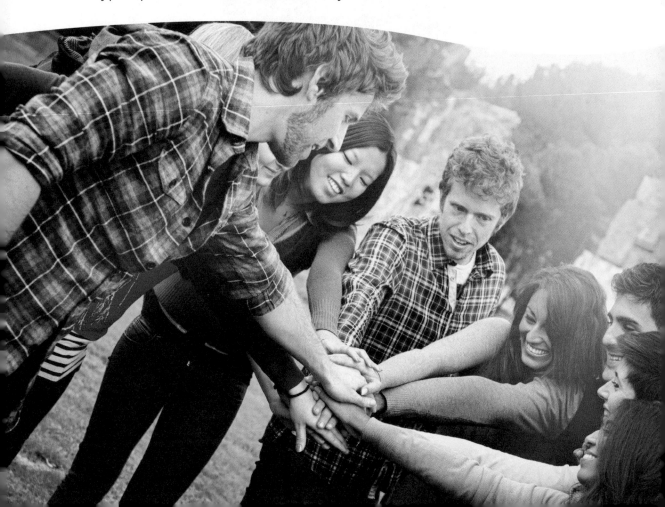

Finally, you'll need some simple group guidelines that outline values and expectations. See the sample in the Appendix and make sure that everyone agrees with and understands those expectations.

When you're finished with these introductory activities, give everyone a chance to respond to these icebreaker questions:

» Use three words to describe how you think about or feel about your body. For example: *limited, beautiful, aging, vulnerable, strong.*

» How do you think God views your body?

LEARNING
TOGETHER

Play the video segment for Session 1. As you watch, use the outline provided to follow along or to take additional notes on anything that stands out to you.

» In Romans 12:1, the apostle Paul says, "Offer your bodies as a *living* sacrifice." Physical discipleship is an ongoing, living sacrifice.

» Paul goes on to say the living sacrifice is "holy and pleasing to God." We're trying to please God with our bodies. We're not trying to please society. What matters is how we look in the eyes of heaven.

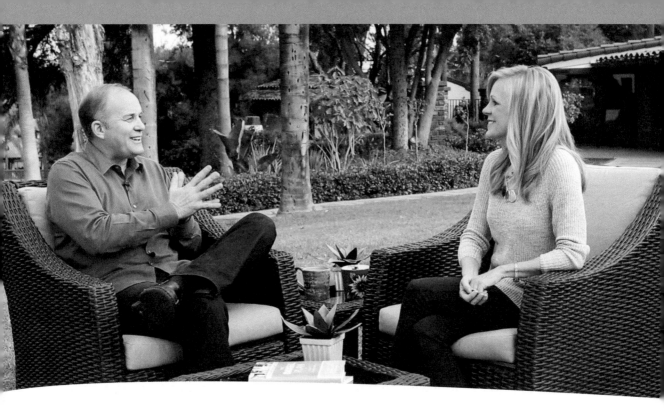

» Our bodies are *instruments* pointing others to God, not *ornaments* pointing to ourselves. We have one body, one tongue, one life, and we want to devote that life to serving and enjoying our Father. We don't need to worry about, "How do I get people to notice and appreciate me?"

» We take care of our bodies so that we have the vitality to speak God's truth, encourage people, hug them, and care for their physical needs.

> *"You are not your own; you were bought at a price.*
> *Therefore honor God with your bodies."*
> 1 Corinthians 6:19–20

» When we believe we own our bodies, we treat them in whatever way we feel comfortable, even abusing them. We treat our bodies differently if we see ourselves as taking care of someone else's property. We treat them with respect and protection.

» God has given us our bodies for a period of time, and we are accountable to him for how we use them. We will give our bodies back to him someday.

> *"For you created my inmost being; you knit me together*
> *in my mother's womb. I praise you because I am*
> *fearfully and wonderfully made; your works*
> *are wonderful, I know that full well."*
> Psalm 139:13–14

» God delights in us, designed us, and knit us together in different bodies for different purposes.

» God looks at us and sees something beautiful that he has made. He doesn't want to see our bodies abused.

» Elton Trueblood said, "Biblical saints aren't good. They're committed." We're going to have bad days, but we are called to be committed overall in our lives to caring for what is God's as an offering of worship.

» We can add a thousand years of service to the kingdom of God if we view our bodies as instruments and we give God another year to use us.

GROWING
TOGETHER

Discuss what you learned from the video. Don't feel obliged to answer every question. Select those that most resonate with your group.

1 Read Romans 12:1 below. What do you think it means to offer your body to God as a living sacrifice? Give some examples of how you might offer your hands to God, your tongue to God, your physical stamina to God.

> *"Therefore, I urge you, brothers and sisters, in view of God's mercy, to offer your bodies as a living sacrifice, holy and pleasing to God— this is your true and proper worship."*
>
> Romans 12:1

2 How have you served God with your body?

3 What's the difference between treating your body as an ornament and treating it as an instrument of God? Give some examples of how you might do each of these things.

4 Read 1 Corinthians 6:19-20 in your Bible or from the notes. How do you react to the idea that your body belongs to God, not to you? Does it surprise you? Did you already know it? Do you resist this idea or embrace it?

5 If your body belongs to God, what are the implications for the way you live?

Read Psalm 139:13 - 14 in your Bible or from the notes. How does it make you feel to know that your body is fearfully and wonderfully made by God? How does that affect the way you view your body?

7 How will Psalm 139 affect the way you treat your body?

══ What I Want ══
to Remember

Complete this activity on your own.

» Briefly review the video outline and any notes you took. Review also any notes from the discussion.

» In the space below, write down the most significant thing you gained from this session—from the video or the discussion. You can share it with the group if you wish.

BETTER
TOGETHER

Now that you've talked about some great ideas, let's get practical—and put what you're learning into action. The Daniel Plan centers around five essential areas of health. In this study you're exploring Faith, so you can begin by identifying one or two steps you can take to have a more vibrant life of faith. Then check out the Food Tip of the Week and the Fitness Move of the Week for some fresh ideas to enrich your journey toward health in those areas. There are also many tips and tools on the danielplan.com website so you can keep growing in all of the Essentials while doing this study. Use or adapt whatever is helpful to you!

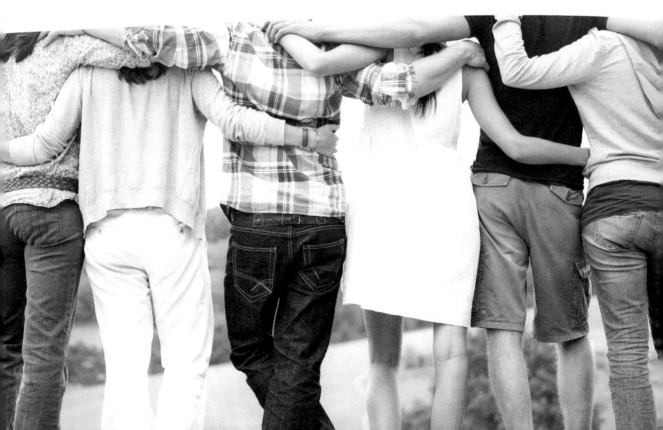

FAITH
Next Steps

Here are a few suggested activities to help you move forward in connecting your body to your faith. Check one or two boxes next to the options you'd like to try this week—choose what works for you.

☐ Lie on the floor with your arms outstretched, or sit comfortably in a chair with your hands on your knees and your palms open upward, or stand with your arms loose at your sides. Close your eyes. Beginning with your feet and moving up your body, offer God the parts of your body as instruments of his righteousness in the world (Romans 6:13). Deliberately give him your feet; ask him to guide you so that your feet take you to places of service, not to places of harm. Give him your legs so that you can stand securely for what is right. If you have mistreated your body, ask for God's forgiveness and the grace to care for your body from now on. Offer your whole self to God as a living sacrifice, holy and pleasing to him. Take your time, asking him to show you how he wants to use your body for his glory.

☐ Spend some time journaling about offering your body as a living sacrifice. Ask yourself if you have any areas of resistance where you don't want to offer your body or some part of your body to God. Do you want your body to belong to you, not to God? Do you want what you eat to be your business, not God's business? Explore your feelings about this in your journal.

☐ Go for a walk out in nature, and have a conversation with God about offering your body to him. Thank him for the way your body moves when you walk. Thank him for your eyes to see beauty around you, for your ears to hear, even your nose to smell.

☐ Pair up with someone in your group who will be your prayer and encouragement partner. Commit to praying for each other's spiritual growth and service to God. Pray that your partner will know how to offer his or her body as a living sacrifice. Plan to send a text of encouragement to your partner during the week. You can also exchange specific prayer requests.

☐ Memorize one of the Bible verses from this session. (A suggested verse for every session is in the Appendix.) Post it someplace you will see it often, and practice repeating it to yourself until you have committed it to memory. When you've memorized one verse, consider taking on this challenge: memorizing one verse during each of the four weeks of this study.

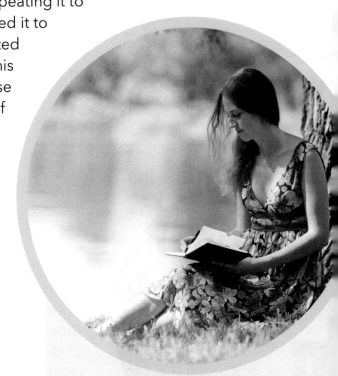

☐ Plan several daily two-minute micro-breaks each day this week. Use that time to thank God for your body and to move your spine and limbs. Or try the Fitness Move of the Week several times a day, using deep breathing and stretching while you praise God for one of his attributes.

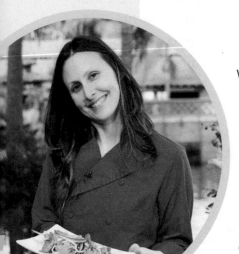

Food Tip
of the Week

Want a quick recipe for adding nutrient-rich foods to a lunch or dinner? This week's spinach salad with fresh orange dressing is loaded with vitamins, minerals, and powerful plant phytonutrients to keep your heart healthy and your brain sharp. Just click the Food Tip of the Week on your video screen (3 minutes), scan the QR code, or go to danielplan.com/foodtip.

Fitness Move
of the Week

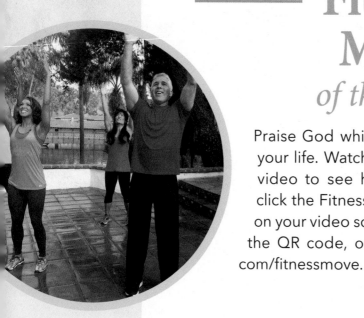

Praise God while you add more movement to your life. Watch the Fitness Move of the Week video to see how it's done. Just click the Fitness Move of the Week on your video screen (1 minute), use the QR code, or go to danielplan.com/fitnessmove.

Praying
Together

Because everything we do in our journey toward health depends on God's power, we end each meeting with prayer and encourage group members to pray for each other during the week.

> *"Rejoice always, pray continually, give thanks in all circumstances; for this is God's will for you in Christ Jesus."*
> 1 Thessalonians 5:16–18

This week, offer a prayer of gratitude to God for your bodies. Take turns offering one- or two-sentence prayers thanking God for something about your body. What parts of your body work well that you tend to take for granted? What are some of the physical gifts God has given you?

Have someone close with this prayer:

Thank you, Lord, for the way you have made our bodies. Thank you for our feet and legs that take us to the people you have called us to serve. Thank you for the way you have designed us to nourish our bodies with food so that we have the energy to love others. Thank you for the arms with which we do work and with which we hug people. Thank you for our hearts that pump blood all over our bodies, and for every vein, artery, and capillary that carries the blood we need. Thank you that your Son Jesus took on a human body just like ours, a body that needed nourishment from food, a body with feet and legs and veins and arteries just like ours. Thank you that he knows just what it's like to live in and through a body, and that he still has a resurrected, glorified body now in heaven. We offer our bodies to you as living sacrifices, holy and pleasing to you. Please do your work in the world through us. I pray this in Jesus' name. Amen.

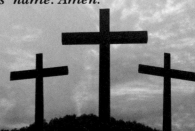

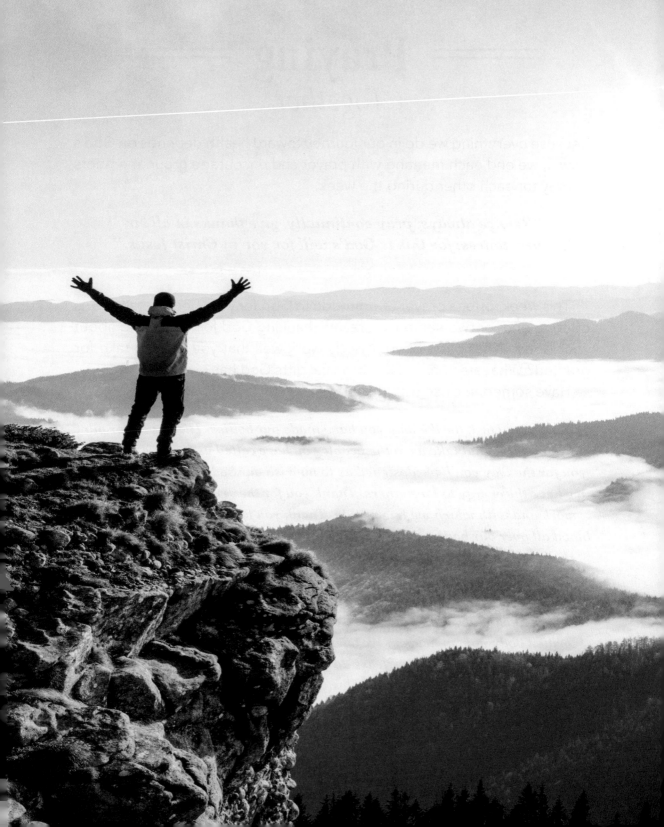

Magnificent Obsession

> "Your kingdom come, your will be
> done, on earth as it is in heaven."
> Matthew 6:10

What is your obsession? What goal gets you out of bed in the morning? What occupies your mind when you're in the shower or standing in line at the store? What do you pursue with passion during the day? What do you think about before you fall asleep at night?

God wants you to be obsessed ... with the right thing. There's something so important to him that he wants it to dominate your schedule. He knows that if you get your top priority straight, the rest of life will follow more easily. So in this session, you'll think about what God wants to be number one on your agenda.

COMING
TOGETHER

The other members of your group can be a huge source of support in sustaining healthy changes in your life. Before watching the video, check in with each other about your experiences since the last session. For example:

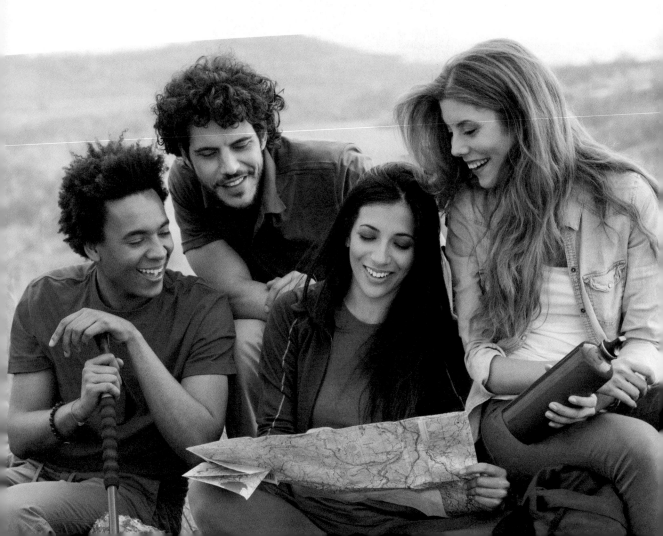

» Briefly share what Next Steps from Session 1 you completed or tried to complete. Were they helpful? If so, how?

» How did Session 1 affect your relationship with God? With your body?

» Have you been practicing The Daniel Plan in other areas, such as Food and Fitness? If so, what have you done? What is working well for you? What questions do you have? What encouragement do you need?

LEARNING
TOGETHER

Play the video segment for Session 2. As you watch, use the outline provided to follow along or to take additional notes on anything that stands out to you.

» In Matthew 6:33, Jesus says, "Seek first [God's] kingdom and his righteousness." That is the magnificent obsession that we are all to pursue.

» In John 6:38, Jesus states the thread that holds his life together: "I have come down from heaven not to do my will but to do the will of him who sent me." A life of surrender, a life of doing the Father's will, is why he came down. That frames his life.

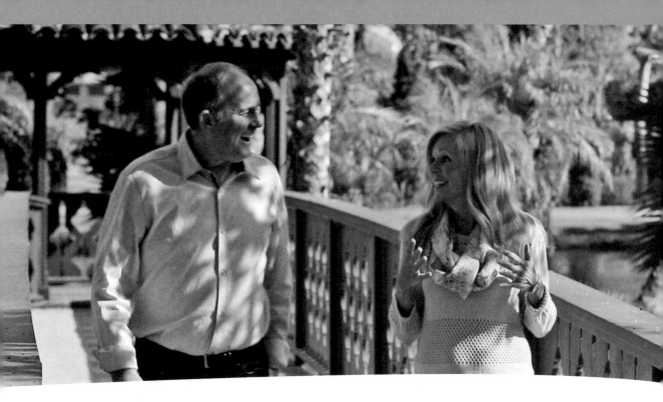

» We are freed from everybody else's expectations so that we can focus on an audience of one: What is God's will for me right now?

» We live our life in chapters. There isn't one mission or one purpose that most of us have for a lifetime. Seeking God's kingdom first is what holds it all together.

» It's freeing to know that God has given us some gifts and not others. We are called to be this, but not that.

» What is your role? Find that role, and be faithful in that role.

> *"Our Lord teaches that the one great secret of the spiritual life is concentration on God and his purposes. Concentration on God is of more value than personal holiness. God can do what he likes with the man who is abandoned to him. God saves us and sanctifies us, then he expects us to concentrate on him in every circumstance we are in."*
> Oswald Chambers

» To concentrate on God, we can ask ourselves every day or two, "What have I done in the last two days that I'll be glad I've done? Have I focused on the right things, so that when my body is laid in the ground, I'll have said they were the right focus and time well spent?"

» We can also ask ourselves, "I have two and a half days left in the week. How do I want to spend those two and a half days so that when my body is in the ground, I'll feel like that was time well spent?"

» We can also listen in the morning, reassess at noon, and evaluate at night. In the morning, we can ask, "Lord, what does it mean to seek first your kingdom today? Does one of my family members need extra care? Do I need to spend some extra time with you to get my heart realigned? Is there someone I'm to reach out to?" Then we can reassess at noon. "How am I doing? Am I being faithful to what you have called me to do?" Then we can evaluate at night. "How did this day go?"

» A lifelong love affair with God gives us the power for living. We don't want to live this life thirsty. If our thirst isn't met by God, then we're trying to get our thirst met by other people instead of loving them.

» When our thirst is met in God—when we know deep down that he's enlisted us, that he loves us, that he's created us, that he's empowering us—then we're finally released to seek first his kingdom and not our own.

GROWING
TOGETHER

Discuss what you learned from the video. Don't feel obliged to answer every question. Select those that most resonate with your group.

 1   What could you do in the next two days that you'll be glad you've done when you're laid in the ground?

"And he died for all, that those who live should no longer live for themselves but for him who died for them and was raised again."

2 Corinthians 5:15

2 The kingdom of God is the realm where God's will is done voluntarily. So, seeking his kingdom first means choosing to do his will. Think about the past day of your life. What do you think was God's will for you to do during the past day? Here are some categories to think about:

» Tasks God wanted you to accomplish

» People God wanted you to treat with love and care

» Time he wanted you to spend with him

» Food, fitness, and the focus of your mind

3 What should we do if we look back on a day and realize that we didn't do the things God had for us to do? Consider, for example, the verses below.

"If we confess our sins, he is faithful and just and will forgive us our sins and purify us from all unrighteousness."
1 John 1:9

"There is no condemnation for those who belong to Christ Jesus."
Romans 8:1 (NLT)

"And I am certain that God, who began the good work within you, will continue his work until it is finally finished on the day when Christ Jesus returns."
Philippians 1:6 (NLT)

4 What if you don't know what God wants you to do? How can you tell the difference between a task God wants you to accomplish and a task you or other people have set that doesn't really matter to him? How would you go about learning to discern the difference?

5 What do you think about the idea of listening in the morning, reassessing at noon, and evaluating your day at night? What would it take for you to make a practice of that?

6 Read Psalm 63:1 below. What do you think it means to get your thirst met by God? How does that work in practical terms?

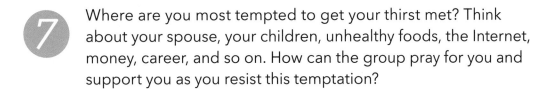

"You, God, are my God, earnestly I seek you; I thirst for you, my whole being longs for you, in a dry and parched land where there is no water."
Psalm 63:1

7 Where are you most tempted to get your thirst met? Think about your spouse, your children, unhealthy foods, the Internet, money, career, and so on. How can the group pray for you and support you as you resist this temptation?

What I Want
to Remember

Complete this activity on your own.

» Briefly review the video outline and any notes you took. Review also any notes from the discussion.

» In the space below, write down the most significant thing you gained from this session—from the video or the discussion. You can share it with the group if you wish.

BETTER
TOGETHER

Now that you've talked about some great ideas, let's get practical — and put what you're learning into action. Begin by identifying one or two steps you can take to have a more vibrant life of faith. Then check out the Food Tip of the Week and the Fitness Move of the Week for some fresh ideas to enrich your journey toward health in those areas. Use or adapt whatever is helpful to you!

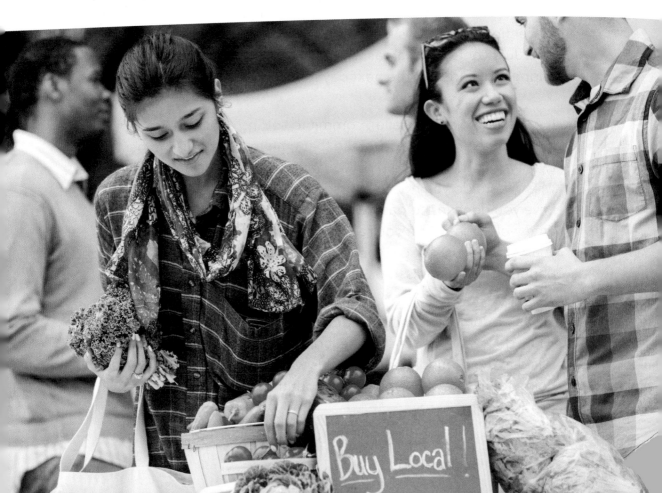

FAITH
Next Steps

Here are a few suggested activities to help you move forward in seeking God's kingdom first. Check one or two boxes next to the options you'd like to try this week—choose what works for you.

☐ Commit to listening in the morning, reassessing at noon, and evaluating at night. In the morning, ask: *Lord, what does it mean for me to seek first your kingdom today?* At noon ask: *How am I doing? Am I being faithful to what you have called me to do?* Before you go to bed, ask: *How did this day go?* Make some notes in a journal so that you can keep track of how things go. Remember: progress, not perfection! Some days may not be good days, and God understands that. Just confess the areas where you fell short, learn from what happened, and start the next day fresh.

☐ If you need to start smaller, commit to setting aside fifteen minutes at the same time each day. Take that time to reflect on the past twenty-four hours. Where do you notice yourself having done God's will? Where do you notice yourself having gotten off track? What have you done in the past twenty-four hours that you'll regard as time well spent when you're laid in the ground? Be gentle with yourself, and just notice. Keep some notes so that you can recognize patterns. Confess missteps and trust in God's forgiveness.

☐ Set aside some time in the middle of the week and ask yourself, "How do I want to spend the rest of this week so that when my body is laid in the ground I can know this was time well spent?" Consider going for a walk while you think about this.

☐ Ask your buddy from your group to encourage you to get your thirst met from God this week. Pray for each other daily. Send each other encouraging texts. You can also check-in midweek and talk about the opportunities you've had to seek God's kingdom first and what you've done with those opportunities.

☐ Commit Matthew 6:33 to memory. You can find it with the memory verses in the Appendix. Post it someplace where you will see it often, and practice repeating it to yourself until you have memorized it.

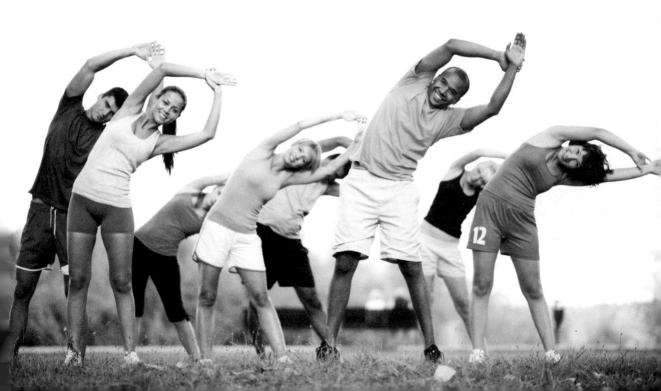

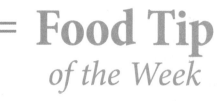

Food Tip
of the Week

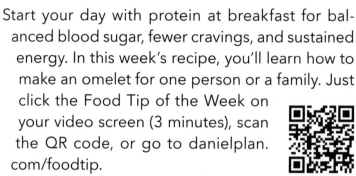

Start your day with protein at breakfast for balanced blood sugar, fewer cravings, and sustained energy. In this week's recipe, you'll learn how to make an omelet for one person or a family. Just click the Food Tip of the Week on your video screen (3 minutes), scan the QR code, or go to danielplan.com/foodtip.

Fitness Move
of the Week

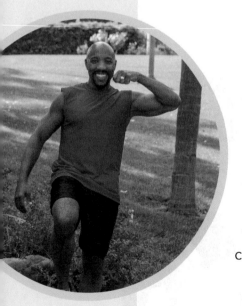

This week, practice gratitude to God while you strengthen your legs and core muscles. Watch this week's move to see how. Just click the Fitness Move of the Week on your video screen (1 minute), use the QR code, or go to danielplan.com/fitnessmove.

Praying
Together

Because everything we do in our journey toward health depends on God's power, we end each meeting with prayer and encourage group members to pray for each other during the week.

Get into smaller groups of two or three people. Share specific needs with your partners, such as questions about God's will in a particular area that you would like God to make clear. Then begin your prayer time by praying aloud together Psalm 63:1:

> *"You, God, are my God, earnestly I seek you; I thirst for you, my whole being longs for you, in a dry and parched land where there is no water."*

Pray for your partners' needs. Pray that they will be able to go to God with their thirst this week and discern his will each day. Even a couple of sentences of prayer are fine if you're not used to praying aloud.

After you've prayed in smaller groups, have someone close with this prayer:

Father, we are thirsty people, and you are the only true source of living water to quench our thirst. We need your help to go to you, and you alone, for our deepest needs. Thank you that you meet our needs partly through your people who care for and support us. We also want to seek your kingdom first. We want to know and do your will. Please open our eyes and ears to discern what you want us to do each day this week. I pray this in Jesus' name. Amen.

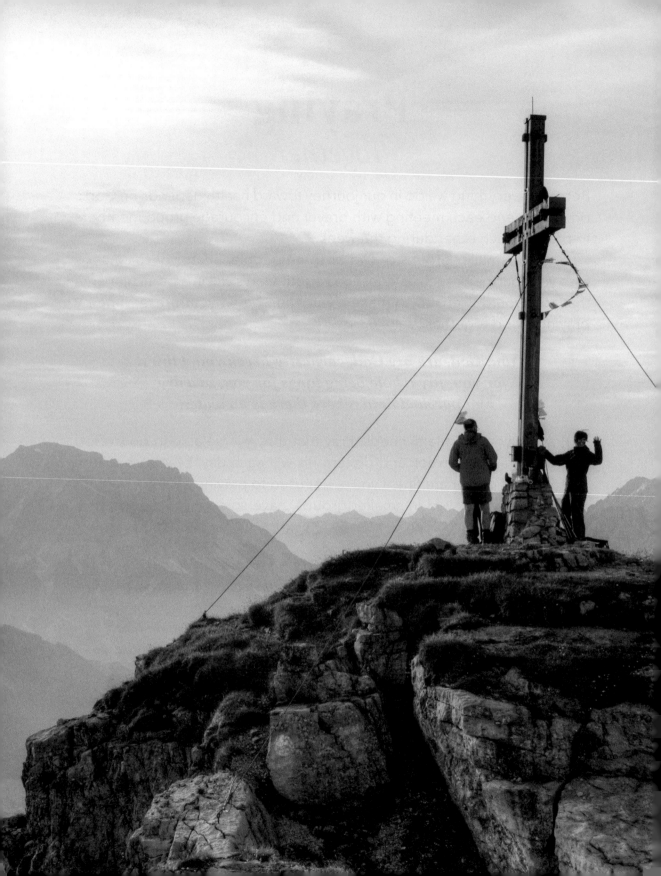

God's Power, Not Willpower

> "And I pray that you, being rooted and established in love, may have power, together with all the Lord's holy people, to grasp how wide and long and high and deep is the love of Christ, and to know this love that surpasses knowledge – that you may be filled to the measure of all the fullness of God."
>
> Ephesians 3:17 – 19

Offering our bodies to God as living sacrifices and seeking his kingdom first aren't easy things to do hour by hour, day after day. We aren't going to create healthy habits by sheer willpower. In fact, while some healthy habits may come naturally to us, we're not going to create good habits in any of our difficult areas on our own. God wants us to put in the effort and come to the end of our resources so that we turn to him. He is eager to empower us whenever we are ready to depend on him. In this session we'll learn how to make a habit of depending on God's power rather than willpower.

COMING
TOGETHER

Before watching the video, check in with each other about your experiences since the last session. For example:

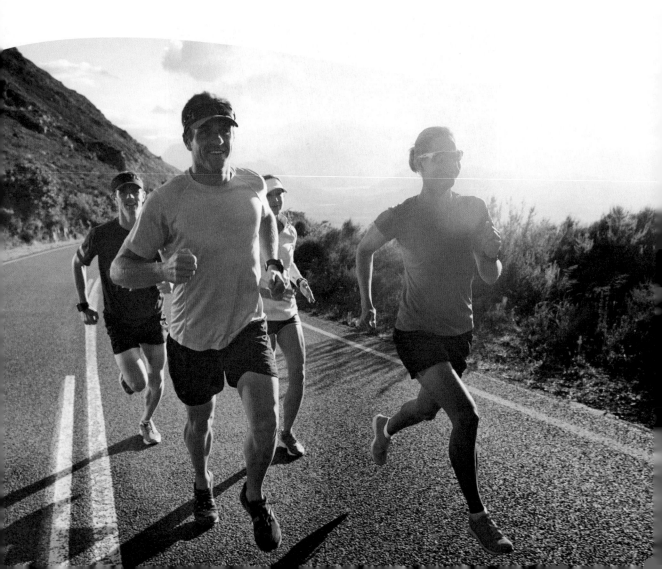

» Briefly share what Next Steps from Session 2 you completed or tried to complete. Were they helpful? If so, how?

» How did Session 2 affect your relationship with God? With other people?

» Have you been practicing The Daniel Plan in other areas, such as Food and Fitness? If so, what have you done? What is working well for you? What questions do you have? What encouragement do you need?

LEARNING
TOGETHER

Play the video segment for Session 3. As you watch, use the outline provided to follow along or to take additional notes on anything that stands out to you.

> *"Be filled with the Spirit."*
> Ephesians 5:18

» Being filled with the Holy Spirit is like running on a cruise ship. We still labor and sweat, but we're carried along by God's Spirit so we can go farther and faster than we could dream of going on our own.

» Literally, in Ephesians 5:18 Paul is saying, "Let yourself be continually filled with the Spirit." We have to do something. We're given an imperative: "Let this happen to you." But it happens to us. We're not making it happen. And it's continuing to happen. So it's really learning a life of continual reliance on God, choosing to let him fill us.

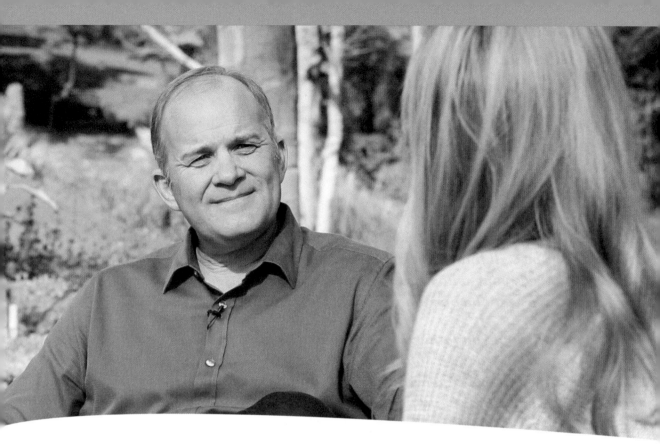

» God says, "If you need to learn dependence on me, I'm going to let you fail. I'm going to let you fall on your face until you really believe you can't do it on your own."

» Victory is found in admitting that we can't get victory on our own. But God can shine through us.

» Jesus tells us to ask God to fill us with the Spirit.

> *"So I say to you: Ask and it will be given to you; seek and you will find; knock and the door will be opened to you. For everyone who asks receives; the one who seeks finds; and to the one who knocks, the door will be opened.*
>
> *"Which of you fathers, if your son asks for a fish, will give him a snake instead? Or if he asks for an egg, will give him a scorpion? If you then, though you are evil, know how to give good gifts to your children, how much more will your Father in heaven give the Holy Spirit to those who ask him!"*
>
> Luke 11:9-13

» Next, we have to believe that if we ask God, he will meet the need. We say to God, "I believe you have called me to do this, so I'm not going to wait around. You said I could ask and have faith in your answer." Then we believe in him and go and do what he's given us to do.

"Therefore I tell you, whatever you ask for in prayer, believe that you have received it, and it will be yours."

Mark 11:24

» Finally, we learn to live in the habit of asking God and believing that he will give the Spirit. We don't just ask occasionally. We ask routinely.

» In every issue we face, we need to consciously surrender to the Spirit. We need to keep asking, keep surrendering, so that it becomes a habit. It's an ongoing dialogue throughout the day as things come up: we connect with God and then take the step of reliance.

> *"I pray that ... he may strengthen you with power through his Spirit in your inner being, so that Christ may dwell in your hearts through faith."*
> Ephesians 3:16 - 17

» The Holy Spirit wants to turn our souls into eyes that are fixed on Jesus.

» The Holy Spirit points to Christ's sufficiency in the cross. It's easy, left to ourselves, to dwell on some issue in our lives. The Holy Spirit says, "Those are issues that God is dealing with, but lift up your head. Look at the cross. Dwell in Jesus." He is the Spirit of worship, helping us to dwell in Christ.

> *"I keep asking that the God of our Lord Jesus Christ, the glorious Father, may give you the Spirit of wisdom and revelation, so that you may know him better. I pray that the eyes of your heart may be enlightened in order that you may know ... his incomparably great power for us who believe."*
> Ephesians 1:17–19

» As our soul's eye is focused on Christ and on his power, he lovingly comes alongside and helps us work through issues. We don't have to push down our emotions. Instead, we go to God with all of who we are and he meets us there.

» John Calvin said, "Once we are in Christ, God doesn't look at our sin and struggle as a prosecuting judge. He looks at it as a physician." How can he help cure? How can he help us get over it?

» When we fail, being filled with the Spirit doesn't mean, "Lord, I promise I'll try harder." It means, "Lord, why did I fail? What was the motivation? What set me up?" Then we wait for God to use our mind to say, "Well, see how you did this, or maybe you pushed this, or maybe it was shame." God is our partner in overcoming the struggle. The Spirit is our Counselor and Comforter.

» We need to know that in the struggle we are deeply loved.

GROWING
TOGETHER

Discuss what you learned from the video. Don't feel obliged to answer every question. Select those that most resonate with your group.

 How would you explain what it means to be filled with the Spirit?

 What do we need to do if we want to be filled with the Spirit to do something? What is for us to do, and what is for God to do?

3 Read 1 Timothy 4:10 below. Are you surprised that you still have to work hard and struggle even while depending on God's Spirit? Why might someone be surprised by that? Why is it necessary to be intentional and dedicated?

> *"This is why we work hard and continue to struggle, for our hope is in the living God, who is the Savior of all people and particularly of all believers."*
> 1 Timothy 4:10 (NLT)

4 What role do our failures play in the process of learning to depend on God's Spirit? Why do you think God doesn't make it all work perfectly right away?

5 Have you ever gone to the Lord after a failure and said, "Lord, why did I fail? What was my motivation in that situation? What set me up for failure?" If so, what happened? If not, what do you expect would happen if you did?

6 How would you put into practice these insights about being filled with the Spirit as you pursue The Daniel Plan? Or as you address some issue in your life?

7 Which of the Scripture passages cited in the "Learning Together" section do you most need to take to heart? Why does it stand out to you?

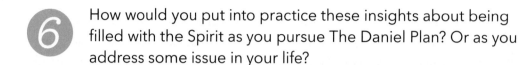

What I Want
to Remember

Complete this activity on your own.

» Briefly review the video outline and any notes you took. Review also any notes from the discussion.

» In the space below, write down the most significant thing you gained from this session—from the video or the discussion. You can share it with the group if you wish.

BETTER
TOGETHER

Now that you've talked about some great ideas, let's get practical—and put what you're learning into action. Begin by identifying one or two steps you can take to have a more vibrant life of faith. Then check out the Food Tip of the Week and the Fitness Move of the Week for some fresh ideas to enrich your journey toward health in those areas. Use or adapt whatever is helpful to you!

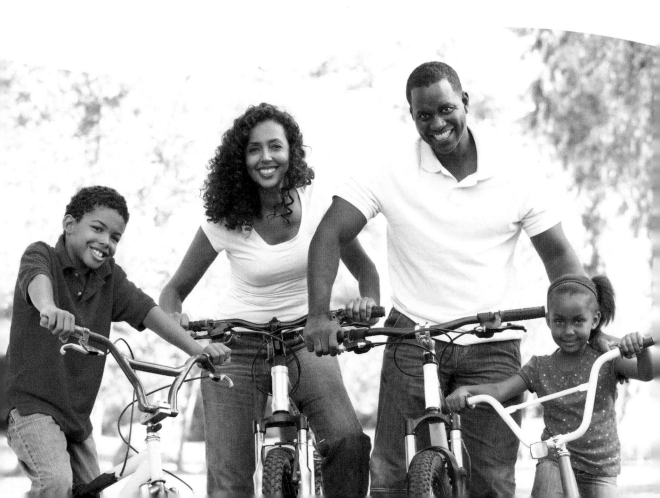

FAITH
Next Steps

Here are a few suggested activities to help you develop a habit of seeking to be filled with the Spirit. Check one or two boxes next to the options you'd like to try this week—choose what works for you.

☐ Post "Be filled with the Spirit (Ephesians 5:18)" somewhere you will see it regularly through the day. Use it as a reminder to pause and ask God to fill you with his Spirit to do whatever task is before you. (You can find the memory verse for the week in the Appendix.)

☐ As you're praying in the morning, ask God to fill you with his Spirit of wisdom and revelation so that you'll *know* his will and with his Spirit of power so that you'll be able to *do* his will.

☐ Use a moment of failure this week as an opportunity to turn to the Spirit as your Counselor. Ask him, "Lord, why did I fail? What was my motivation in that moment? What set me up for failure?" Then take some time to listen and think. It may help if you write down your thoughts. You could include this conversation in your before-bed review of your day.

☐ Connect with your buddy this week and encourage each other to pray to be filled with the Spirit.

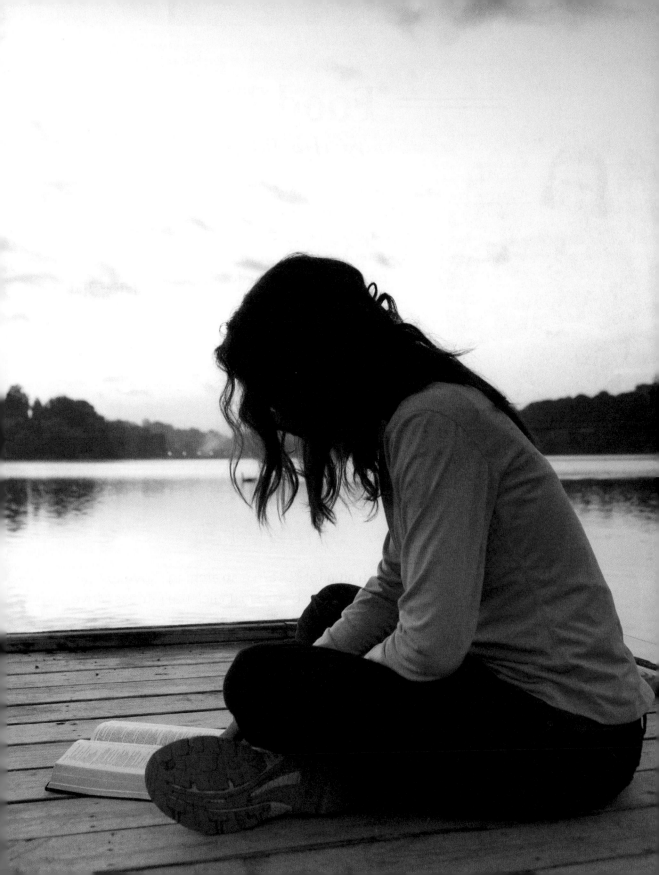

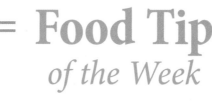

Food Tip
of the Week

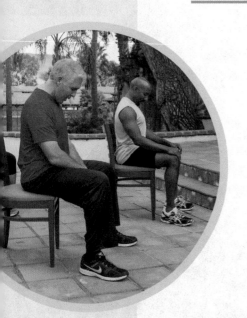

To "eat the rainbow," fill your shopping cart with vibrant colors from across the spectrum. Be open to experimenting, trying colorful new fruits and vegetables, because where there is color, there is powerful nutrition for healthy, Daniel Plan living. Just click the Food Tip of the Week on your video screen (3 minutes), scan the QR code, or go to danielplan.com/foodtip.

Fitness Move
of the Week

Do you sit a lot? Learn a stretching move to melt and relax your body. Just click the Fitness Move of the Week on your video screen (1 minute), use the QR code, or go to danielplan.com/fitnessmove.

Praying
Together

Because everything we do in our journey toward health depends on God's power, we end each meeting with prayer and encourage group members to pray for each other during the week.

Let everyone offer up one-sentence prayers that begin like this: "Lord, please fill me with your Spirit to _____." Have someone close with this prayer:

Lord, thank you for your Holy Spirit. He is the Spirit of wisdom and revelation. He is the Holy Spirit who wants to empower us to be holy. He is our Counselor and Comforter. He is your gift to us, your presence in us. Please remind us to ask to be filled with your Spirit throughout the coming days, and please give us the faith to believe you are answering that prayer. Please remind us of your love in our struggles. I pray this in Jesus' name. Amen.

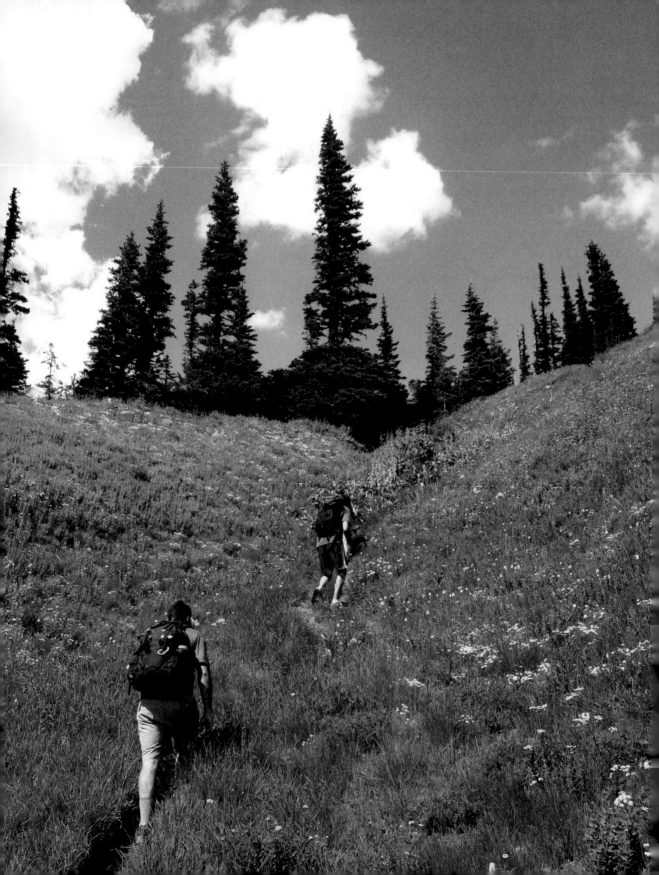

Your Soul's Path to God

> "Show me your ways, LORD,
> teach me your paths."
> Psalm 25:4

Sometimes we look at someone else's spiritual life and feel that we should be just like them. Maybe we feel we should be as lively in worship services as they are, or as good at spending an hour alone with God as they are, or as active in taking meals to the sick as they are. Yet while these are all good practices, the truth is that there is no one-size-fits-all way to draw closer to God. He has designed us with different temperaments intended to relate to him in different ways. In this session we'll look at nine different pathways to going deep with God.

COMING
TOGETHER

Before watching the video, check in with each other about your experiences since the last session. For example:

» Briefly share what Next Steps from Session 3 you completed or tried to complete. Were they helpful? If so, how?

» How did Session 3 affect your relationship with God? How did it affect your ability to do God's will with the Spirit's help?

» Have you been practicing The Daniel Plan in other areas, such as Food and Fitness? If so, what have you done? What is working well for you? What questions do you have? What encouragement do you need?

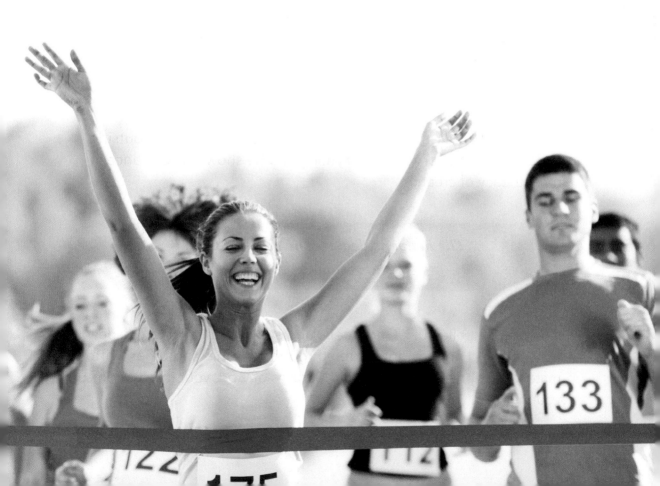

LEARNING
TOGETHER

Play the video segment for Session 4. As you watch, use the outline provided to follow along or to take additional notes on anything that stands out to you.

» If we can find a way of relating to God that we look forward to—that makes us feel like we've missed something if we haven't met with God like that—then we'll be far more likely to spend more time with God. In the Scriptures, there are myriad ways that people relate to the same God.

» If you're a Naturalist, your heart is opened up when you get outside, because God has ordered everything and he shows his brilliance in the intricacy of creation.

> *"The heavens declare the glory of God."*
> Psalm 19:1

» If you're an Intellectual, God opens up your heart by giving you new concepts and new insights, often through the Bible and other written material. When you think about the truths of God, your mind opens up your heart.

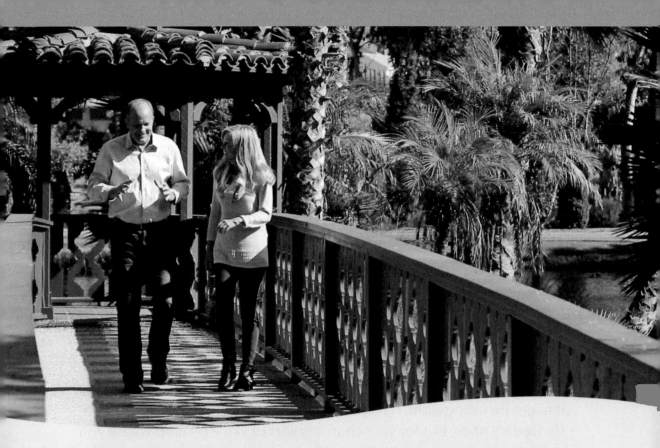

"Now the Berean Jews were of more noble character than those in Thessalonica, for they received the message with great eagerness and examined the Scriptures every day to see if what Paul said was true."

Acts 17:11

» If you're an Ascetic, you like to get away because you don't want distractions. You like to be alone. Because you live in an interior world, a lot of artsy stuff or noise will take you away from the presence of God.

"At daybreak, Jesus went out to a solitary place."

Luke 4:42

» If you're a Sensate, on the other hand, your senses lead you into God's presence. You may like architecture—you go into a cathedral and there is something that just floods your soul. You like majestic music. Maybe you like icons or a cross or other visual aids that turn your thoughts to God. Maybe you even like smells.

> *"Make the tabernacle with ten curtains of finely twisted linen and blue, purple and scarlet yarn, with cherubim woven into them by a skilled worker."*
>
> Exodus 26:1

» If you're an Activist, your soul is awakened in the midst of confrontation. It might be evangelism, it might be a social cause where you stand up for God's justice, but for you, church is sort of like a pit stop where you get volunteers and you get filled up to take risks in God's name.

> *"In the temple courts [Jesus] found people selling cattle, sheep and doves, and others sitting at tables exchanging money. So he made a whip out of cords, and drove all from the temple courts, both sheep and cattle; he scattered the coins of the money changers and overturned their tables."*
>
> John 2:14-15

» If you're a Caregiver, your soul is awakened to God when you're giving care to someone in need.

"Then the righteous will answer him, 'Lord, when did we see you hungry and feed you, or thirsty and give you something to drink? When did we see you a stranger and invite you in, or needing clothes and clothe you? When did we see you sick or in prison and go to visit you?'

"The King will reply, 'Truly I tell you, whatever you did for one of the least of these brothers and sisters of mine, you did for me.'"

Matthew 25:37–40

» If you're a Contemplative, you think of God as your loving Father, Bridegroom, and Friend. You're less interested in accomplishing great things for him than in sitting with him and loving him with the purest love imaginable.

> *"I belong to my beloved, and his desire is for me."*
> Song of Songs 7:10

» If you're an Enthusiast, you're inspired by joyful celebration. You want to be with other Christians clapping your hands and shouting "Amen!" You don't want to just know truths; you want to experience them.

"Clap your hands, all you nations;
shout to God with cries of joy."

Psalm 47:1

» If you're a Traditionalist, rituals and symbols speak to you. You're drawn to historic expressions of faith. For you, a centuries-old prayer has depth and special meaning.

"Come, let us bow down in worship,
let us kneel before the LORD our Maker."
Psalm 95:6

» You don't have to follow all nine pathways, you don't have to be like someone else—they have their walk with God, but God wants a unique relationship with you.

"For the eyes of the LORD range throughout
the earth to strengthen those whose hearts
are fully committed to him."
2 Chronicles 16:9

» God is looking on. He is looking for people who say, "Okay, this is my life. I'm going to dedicate it to him." God is searching us out to strengthen us and invite us into his work.

» When we can find a way to spend more time in God's presence, it shapes us. It changes our souls, our desires. Obedience flows from there. It becomes a lifelong love affair of worship and devotion, where we're satisfied and transformed.

GROWING
TOGETHER

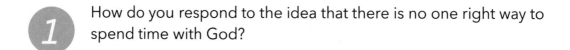

Discuss what you learned from the video. Don't feel obliged to answer every question. Select those that most resonate with your group.

1 How do you respond to the idea that there is no one right way to spend time with God?

2 Reread the descriptions of the nine spiritual pathways in the "Learning Together" section. Which pathways most appeal to you? Why? (If you have time in your meeting, allow ten minutes for everyone to complete the inventory in the "FAITH Next Steps" section. Then discuss your results.)

3 How can you use your knowledge of your spiritual temperament to design time with God that you will want to pursue? Review the list of ideas after the inventory in "FAITH Next Steps," or come up with your own ideas. As a group, help each person make a plan. Some of you may want to team up to pursue something together, while others will prefer to have solitary time with God.

4 What challenges do you face in planning consistent time with God in ways that fit your spiritual temperament? How can the group pray for you?

5 How can you address those challenges? What help do you need?

6 Why is it important to value the different ways God has created each person to interact with him?

7 What are the most valuable things you have gotten out of this study of Faith? What will you take with you? How has the group helped you?

What I Want
to Remember

Complete this activity on your own.

» Briefly review the video outline and any notes you took. Review also any notes from the discussion.

» In the space below, write down the most significant thing you gained from this session—from the video or the discussion. You can share it with the group if you wish.

BETTER
TOGETHER

Now that you've talked about some great ideas, let's get practical — and put what you're learning into action. Begin by identifying one or two steps you can take to have a more vibrant life of faith. Then check out the Food Tip of the Week and the Fitness Move of the Week for some fresh ideas to enrich your journey toward health in those areas. Use or adapt whatever is helpful to you!

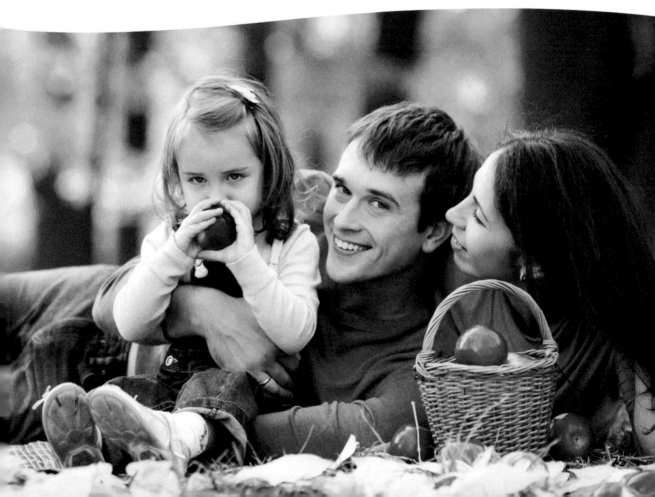

FAITH
Next Steps

To help you move forward in understanding and living by your spiritual temperament, take the following inventory on your own from the book *Sacred Pathways* by Gary Thomas. After you finish it, choose one or two of the next steps that fit your temperament.

For each item below, rate yourself from 1–5, with 5 being very true and 1 being not true at all. Record your answer in the space provided.

THE NATURALIST

_____ 1. I feel closest to God when I'm surrounded by what he has made – the mountains, the forests, or the sea.

_____ 2. I feel cut off if I have to spend too much time indoors, just listening to speakers or singing songs. Nothing makes me feel closer to God than being outside.

_____ 3. I would prefer to spend an hour beside a small brook rather than be involved in a group service.

_____ 4. If I could escape to a garden to pray on a cold day, walk through a meadow on a warm day, and take a trip by myself to the mountains on another day, I would be very happy. (On a scale of 5 [very happy] to 1 [bored].)

_____ 5. A book called *Nature's Sanctuaries: A Picture Book* would be appealing to me.

_____ 6. Seeing God's beauty in nature is more moving to me than understanding new concepts, participating in a formal religious service, or participating in social causes.

_____ *The total of all of your answers for items 1 through 6.*

THE SENSATE

_____ 7. I feel closest to God when I'm in a church that allows my senses to come alive — when I can see, smell, hear, and almost taste his majesty.

_____ 8. I enjoy attending a "high church" service with incense and formal Communion or Eucharist.

_____ 9. I'd have a difficult time worshiping in a church building that is plain and lacks a sense of awe or majesty. Beauty is very important to me, and I have a difficult time putting up with second-rate Christian art or music.

_____ 10. The words *sensuous*, *colorful*, and *aromatic* are very appealing to me.

_____ 11. A book called *The Beauty of Worship* would be appealing to me.

_____ 12. I would really enjoy using drawing exercises or art to improve my prayer life.

_____ *The total of all of your answers for items 7 through 12.*

THE TRADITIONALIST

_____ 13. I feel closest to God when I'm participating in a familiar form of worship that has memories dating back to my childhood. Rituals and traditions move me more than anything else.

_____ 14. Individualism within the church is a real danger. Christianity is a corporate faith, and most of our worship should have a corporate expression.

_____ 15. The words *tradition* and *history* are very appealing to me.

_____ 16. Participating in a formal liturgy or prayer book service; developing symbols that I could place in my car, home, or office; and developing a Christian calendar for our family to follow are activities that I would enjoy.

_____ 17. A book titled *Symbolism and Liturgy in Worship* would be appealing to me.

_____ 18. I would really enjoy developing a personal rule (or ritual) of prayer.

_____ *The total of all of your answers for items 13 through 18.*

THE ASCETIC

_____ 19. I feel closest to God when I am alone and there is nothing to distract me from focusing on his presence.

_____ 20. I don't mind worshiping God in a group, but I'd much prefer to be alone.

_____ 21. The words *silence*, *solitude*, and *discipline* are very appealing to me.

_____ 22. Taking an overnight retreat by myself at a monastery, where I could spend large amounts of time alone in a small room; praying to God and studying his Word; and fasting for one or more days are all activities I would enjoy.

_____ 23. I would enjoy reading the book *A Place Apart: Monastic Prayer and Practice for Everyone* by M. Basil Pennington.

_____ 24. I would really enjoy spending two hours alone in silent prayer in a small, white room.

_____ *The total of all of your answers for items 19 through 24.*

THE ACTIVIST

_____ 25. I feel closest to God when I'm cooperating with him in standing up for his justice: writing letters to government officials and newspaper editors, picketing at an abortion clinic, urging people to vote, or becoming familiar with current issues.

_____ 26. I get very frustrated if I see apathetic Christians who don't become active. I want to drop everything else I'm doing and help the church overcome its apathy.

_____ 27. The words *courageous confrontation* and *social activism* are very appealing to me.

_____ 28. Confronting a social evil, attending a meeting to challenge the new curriculum before the local school board, and volunteering on a political campaign are activities that are important to me.

_____ 29. The book written by Frank Schaeffer, *A Time for Anger*, would be an important book for me to read.

_____ 30. I would like to awaken the church from its apathy.

_____ *The total of all of your answers for items 25 through 30.*

THE CAREGIVER

_____ 31. I feel closest to God when I see him in the needy, the poor, the sick, and the imprisoned. I feel God's presence most strongly when I am sitting quietly beside the bed of someone who is lonely or ill or taking a meal to someone in need. You can count on me to offer a ride or volunteer for helping activities.

_____ 32. I grow weary of Christians who spend their time singing songs while a sick neighbor goes without a hot meal or a family in need doesn't get help fixing their car.

_____ 33. The words *service* and *compassion* are very appealing to me.

_____ 34. I sense God's power when I am counseling a friend who has lost his job, preparing meals for or fixing the car of a family in need, and spending a week at an orphanage in Mexico.

_____ 35. A book like *The Counsel of a Friend* by Lynda Elliot would be very appealing to me.

_____ 36. I would rather nurse someone to health or help someone repair their house than teach an adult Sunday school class.

_____ *The total of all of your answers for items 31 through 36.*

THE ENTHUSIAST

_____ 37. I feel closest to God when my heart is sent soaring, and I feel like I want to burst, worship God all day long, and shout out his Name. Celebrating God and his love is my favorite form of worship.

_____ 38. God is an exciting God, and we should be excited about worshiping him. I don't understand how some Christians can say they love God, and then act like they're going to a funeral whenever they walk into church.

_____ 39. The words *celebration* and *joy* are very appealing to me.

_____ 40. I would enjoy attending a workshop on learning to worship through dance or attending several worship sessions with contemporary music. I expect that God is going to move in some unexpected ways.

_____ 41. I would enjoy reading the book *Windows on the Soul: A Look at Dreams and Their Meanings* by Dr. Paul Meier and Dr. Robert Wise.

_____ 42. I enjoy listening to music and worship recordings.

_____ *The total of all of your answers for items 37 through 42.*

THE CONTEMPLATIVE

_____ 43. I feel closest to God when my emotions are awakened; when God quietly touches my heart, tells me that he loves me, and makes me feel like I'm his closest friend. I would rather be alone with God, contemplating his love, than participate in a formal liturgy or be distracted by a walk outside.

_____ 44. The most difficult times in my faith are when I can't feel God's presence within me.

_____ 45. The words *lover*, *intimacy*, and *heart* are very appealing to me.

_____ 46. I really enjoy having thirty minutes of uninterrupted time a day to sit in quiet prayer and "hold hands" with God, writing love letters to him and enjoying his presence.

_____ 47. I would enjoy reading *Transforming Friendship* by James Houston.

_____ 48. When I think of God, I think of love, friendship, and adoration more than anything else.

_____ *The total of all of your answers for items 43 through 48.*

THE INTELLECTUAL

_____ 49. I feel closest to God when I learn something new about him that I didn't understand before. My mind needs to be stimulated. It's very important to me that I know exactly what I believe.

_____ 50. I get frustrated when the church focuses too much on feelings and spiritual experience. Of far more importance is the need to understand the Christian faith and have proper doctrine.

_____ 51. The words *concept* and *truth* are very appealing to me.

_____ 52. I feel close to God when I participate in several hours of uninterrupted study time, reading God's Word, some helpful books, and then perhaps having an opportunity to teach (or participate in a discussion with) a small group.

_____ 53. A book on church dogmatics would be appealing to me.

_____ 54. I spend more money on books than music recordings.

_____ *The total of all of your answers for items 49 through 54.*

SCORING: The highest number of points possible is obviously 30 for each pathway. The higher your score, the stronger the dominance of this spiritual temperament in your life. But most of us have more than one spiritual temperament. Any score of 15 or higher indicates a preference for that temperament.

Look over your scores. List each temperament in order of its importance to your life:

1. _____

2. _____

3. _____

4. _____

5. _____

6. _____

7. _____

8. _____

9. _____

What will you do with this information? Now that you have a better idea of your spiritual temperament, how can you design your spiritual life so that you regularly give your soul what it most craves, while also including some times when you stretch yourself into experiences that don't come most naturally to you? Here are some options to get you started:

- ☐ Get outdoors for a walk, a run, or a bike ride in a natural setting. If you live in an urban setting, find a park, a botanical garden, or even a street lined with large trees. Spend your time there in prayer, thanksgiving, and worship of God as Creator. Notice the details of what he has created, and praise him for those things.

- ☐ If you're a Naturalist but the weather makes it hard for you to be outdoors regularly, try bringing some of nature into the place in your home where you spend time with God. Grow plants in pots. Arrange a collection of pine cones or dried grasses. Get a fish tank.

- ☐ Attend a worship service that ministers to your longing for beauty. If you're drawn to the grand and liturgical, where could you experience that?

- ☐ Visit an art gallery, perhaps one with a collection of classical Christian art, or one with contemporary art whose abstractions will raise your soul to God. As you stand before each piece, praise God for being the source of all beauty. If you don't have access to a gallery, try buying two or three prints of whatever raises your soul, whether that's a photograph of a sunset or a Renaissance painting. Place them in the space where you meet with God.

- ☐ Prayerfully listen to an album of whatever type of music draws you to God, whether that's contemporary Christian music, Bach, or Gregorian chant.

- [ ] Buy a copy of a prayer book, such as *The Book of Common Prayer*. Or google "morning prayer" or "liturgy of the hours" to see traditional rituals of daily prayer. Use these to design your own daily ritual of prayer. A simple option is to pray two or three psalms aloud each day in addition to your own prayers.

- [ ] De-clutter a space where you can spend time alone with God in silence and simplicity.

- [ ] Is there a social or evangelistic mission that God has been calling you to? What is the next step you need to take in following him in that mission?

- [ ] Reach out to someone in need. Take them a meal, offer to babysit their children for an evening, fix something broken in their house, or just offer them a listening ear.

- [ ] Attend a worship celebration with one or more people from your small group. Let yourself be caught up in the worship and enjoy the fellowship afterward.

- [ ] Take your Bible study to the next level. If there is a study resource you have been thinking about getting, this may be the time. Commit to daily study time.

- [ ] Do the Fitness Move of the Week each day while you take your requests to God.

Food Tip
of the Week

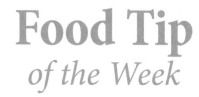

For a jumpstart to healthier eating, check out the 10-day Daniel Plan detox or the 40-day core meal plan. Both plans include the fundamentals of eating the Daniel Plan way, enjoying real, whole, fresh foods while helping you uncover the foods that could be sabotaging your health journey. This week you'll be introduced to one of the many delicious and nutritious recipes in *The Daniel Plan* book. Just click the Food Tip of the Week on your video screen (3 minutes), scan the QR code, or go to danielplan.com/foodtip.

Fitness Move
of the Week

Learn a move you can do while you go to God with your requests each day. Just click the Fitness Move of the Week on your video screen (1 minute), use the QR code, or go to danielplan.com/fitnessmove.

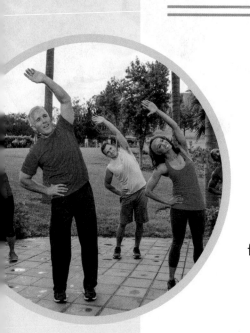

Praying
Together

Because everything we do in our journey toward health depends on God's power, we end each meeting with prayer and encourage group members to pray for each other during the week.

Take turns offering one- or two-sentence prayers expressing things for which you're grateful to God. It might be the ways he has designed you to get to know him—through nature, through celebration, through quiet contemplation, or one of the other pathways. It might be for things you've received in this group. What has God done for you that you're thankful for? And if you still have questions about how to build consistent time with God into your life, offer him your questions and your need for help.

Have someone close with this prayer:

Father, you have designed each of us to relate to you in unique ways. Thank you for revealing yourself to some of us in the natural world you have created. Thank you for ministering to some of us through our senses, and to some of us through centuries-old traditions. Thank you for drawing close to us in silence and solitude, or through boisterous celebration. Thank you for touching some of our hearts through the divine romance and others through truth revealed to our minds. Thank you for those among us who stand up for justice or care for the needy. Please show each of us how to live out the magnificent obsession with seeking your kingdom, with doing your will. We want to build lifelong habits of pursuing you. Please show us how, and fill us with your Holy Spirit to follow through consistently. I pray this in Jesus' name. Amen.

Appendix

Appendix

Group Guidelines

Our goal: To provide a safe environment where participants experience authentic community and spiritual growth.

OUR VALUES	
Group Attendance	To give priority to the group meeting. We will call or email if we will be late or absent.
Safe Environment	To help create a safe place where people can be heard and feel loved.
Respect Differences	To be gentle and gracious to people with different spiritual maturity, personal opinions, or personalities. Remember we are all works in progress!
Confidentiality	To keep anything that is shared strictly confidential and within the group, and to avoid sharing information about those outside the group.
Encouragement for Growth	We want to spiritually multiply our life by serving others with our God-given gifts.
Rotating Hosts/Leaders and Homes	To encourage different people to host the group in their homes, and to rotate the responsibility of facilitating each meeting.

We have found that groups thrive when they talk about expectations up front and come into agreement on some of the following details.

Refreshments/mealtimes _____

Child care _____

When we will meet (day of week) _____

Where we will meet (place) _____

We will begin at (time) _____ and end at _____

We will look for a compatible time to attend a worship service together.

Our primary worship service time will be _____

Leadership 101

Congratulations! You have responded to the call to help shepherd Jesus' flock. There are few other tasks in the family of God that surpass the contribution you will be making. As you prepare to lead, whether it is one session or four, here are a few thoughts to keep in mind. We encourage you to read these and review them with each new discussion leader before he or she leads.

1. **Remember that you are not alone.** God knows everything about you, and he knew that you would be asked to lead your group. It is common for leaders to feel that they are not ready to lead. Moses, Solomon, Jeremiah, Timothy—they all were reluctant to lead. God promises, "Never will I leave you; never will I forsake you" (Hebrews 13:5). You will be blessed as you serve.

2. **Don't try to do it alone.** Pray right now for God to help you build a healthy leadership team. If you can enlist a co-leader to help you lead the group, you will find your experience to be much richer. That person might take half the group in a second discussion circle if your group is as large as ten people or more. Your co-leader might lead the prayer time or handle the hosting tasks, welcoming people and getting them refreshments. This is your chance to involve as many people as you can in building a healthy group. All you have to do is call and ask people to help; you'll be surprised at the response.

3. **Just be yourself.** God wants you to use your unique gifts and temperament. Don't try to do things exactly like another leader; do them in a way that fits you! Just admit it when you don't have an answer, and apologize when you make a mistake. Your group will love you for it, and you'll sleep better at night.

4. **Prepare for your meeting ahead of time.** Review the session, view the video, and write down your responses to each question. If paper and pens are needed, such as for gathering group members' names and email addresses (see "Coming Together" in Session 1), be sure you have the necessary supplies. Think about which "Next Steps" you will do.

   If you're leading Session 1, look over the Group Guidelines and be ready to review them with the group. If child care will be an issue for your group, for example, be prepared to talk about options. Some groups have the adults share the cost of a babysitter (or two) to care for children in a different part of the house where the adults are meeting. Other groups use one home for the kids and another for the adults. A third idea is to rotate the responsibility of caring for the children in the same home or one nearby.

5. **Pray for your group members by name.** Before you begin your session, go around the room in your mind and pray for each member. You may want to review the group's prayer list at least once a week. Ask God to use your time together to work in the heart of each person uniquely. Expect God to lead you to whomever he wants you to encourage or challenge in a special way.

6. **When you ask a question, be patient.** Read each question aloud and wait for someone to respond. Sometimes people need a moment or two of silence to think about the question, and if silence doesn't bother you, it won't bother anyone else. After someone responds, affirm the response with a simple "thanks" or "good job." Then ask, "How about somebody else?" or "Would someone who hasn't shared like to add anything?" Be sensitive to new people or reluctant members who aren't ready to participate yet. If you give them a safe setting, they will open up over time. Don't go around the circle and have everyone answer every question. Your goal is a conversation in which the group members talk to each other in a natural way.

7. **Break up into small groups each week or people won't stay.** If your group has more than eight people, we strongly encourage you to have the group gather sometimes in discussion circles of three or four people during the "Growing Together" section of the study. With a greater opportunity to talk in a small circle, people will connect more with the study, apply more quickly what they are learning, and ultimately get more out of it. A small circle also encourages a quiet person to participate and tends to minimize the effect of a more vocal or dominant member. It can also help people feel more loved in your group. When you gather again at the end of the section, you can have one person summarize the highlights from each circle.

    Small circles are also helpful during prayer time. People who are not accustomed to praying aloud will feel more comfortable trying it with just two or three others. Also, prayer requests won't take as much time, so circles will have more time to actually pray. When you gather back with the whole group, you can have one person from each circle briefly update everyone on the prayer requests.

8. **One final challenge for new leaders:** Before your opportunity to lead, look up each of the four passages listed below. Read each one as a devotional exercise to help equip you with a shepherd's heart. If you do this, you will be more than ready for your first meeting.

    Matthew 9:36
    1 Peter 5:2–4
    Psalm 23
    Ezekiel 34:11–16

For additional tips and resources, go to danielplan.com/tools.

Memory Verses

SESSION 1

"Therefore, I urge you, brothers and sisters, in view of God's mercy, to offer your bodies as a living sacrifice, holy and pleasing to God — this is your true and proper worship."

Romans 12:1

SESSION 2

"Seek first [God's] kingdom and his righteousness, and all these things will be given to you as well."

Matthew 6:33

SESSION 3

"Be filled with the Spirit."

Ephesians 5:18

SESSION 4

"For the eyes of the LORD range throughout the earth to strengthen those whose hearts are fully committed to him."

2 Chronicles 16:9

About the Contributors

GUEST SPEAKERS

Gary Thomas is a bestselling author and international speaker whose ministry brings people closer to Christ and closer to others. He unites the study of Scripture, church history, and the Christian classics to foster spiritual growth and deeper relationships within the Christian community. Church leaders and pastors appreciate Gary's ability to challenge and encourage the spiritual depth of an audience.

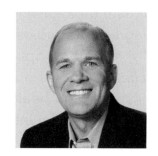

Dee Eastman is the Founding Director of The Daniel Plan that has helped over 15,000 people lose 260,000 pounds in the first year alone. Dee completed her education in Health Science with an emphasis in long-term lifestyle change. Her experience in corporate wellness and ministry has fueled her passion to help people transform their health while drawing closer to God. She coauthored the *Doing Life Together* Bible study series and was a contributing author of *The Daniel Plan*.

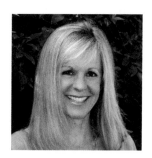

SIGNATURE CHEFS

Sally Cameron is a professional chef, author, recipe developer, educator, certified health coach, and one of the contributors to *The Daniel Plan Cookbook*. Sally's passion is to inspire people to create great-tasting meals at home using healthy ingredients and easy techniques. Sally is the publisher of the popular food blog, *A Food Centric Life*. She holds a culinary degree from The Art Institute and health coaching certification from The Institute for Integrative Nutrition.

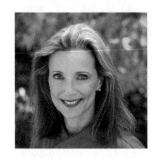

Jenny Ross is the internationally recognized chef, author, educator, and force behind Jenny Ross Living Foods, including the raw food restaurant 118 Degrees, the popular Raw Basics detox meal programs, and nationwide grocery product line 118 Degrees. She has been an early pioneer of the raw movement, coaching clients about the healing power of living foods, while motivating them to adopt a more vibrant, healthy lifestyle. She has a degree in holistic nutrition and certificates as a health and life coach. Jenny was one of the contributing chefs of *The Daniel Plan Cookbook*.

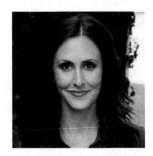

Mareya Ibrahim is best known as "The Fit Foodie." She is an award-winning entrepreneur, television chef, author, and one of The Daniel Plan signature chefs. She is also the CEO and founder of Grow Green Industries, Inc. and cocreator of eatCleaner, the premier lifestyle destination for fit food information. Her book *The Clean Eating Handbook* is touted as the "go-to" guide for anyone looking to eat cleaner and get leaner. She is a featured chef on ABC's Emmy-nominated cooking show *Recipe Rehab,* eHow.com, and Livestrong, and the food expert for San Diego's Channel 6 News.

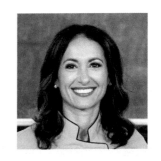

Robert Sturm is one of California's premier chefs and food designers. He has been in the food service industry for more than thirty years, working as an independent consultant to leading restaurant chains around the country. He has been featured in many publications, appears on television and radio, and has been a featured chef at the United Nations, the White House, and the Kremlin. Robert is the three-time winner of the U.S. Chef's Open, a past gold medal member of the U.S. Culinary Olympic Team, and has won many national and international culinary titles and food design awards.

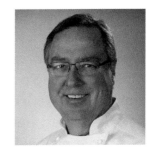

FITNESS TEAM

Sean Foy is an internationally renowned authority on fitness, weight management, and healthy living. As an author, exercise physiologist, behavioral coach, and speaker, Sean has earned the reputation as "America's Fast Fitness Expert." With an upbeat and sensible approach to making fitness happen, he's taken the message of "simple moves" fitness all over the world. Sean is the author of *Fitness That Works, Walking 4 Wellness, The Burst Workout,* and a contributing author *The Daniel Plan.*

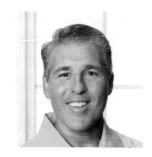

Basheerah Ahmad is a well-known celebrity fitness expert, with a heart for serving God's people. Whether it be through television appearances (*Dr. Phil, The Doctors*), writing fitness and nutrition books, speaking publicly about health, or teaching classes in under-served communities, Basheerah has dedicated her life to improving the health of people everywhere. She has a MS in Exercise Science and numerous certifications in fitness and nutrition. She was a lead fitness instructor for *The Daniel Plan in Action* fitness video series.

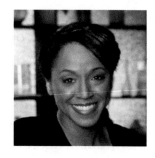

Tony "The Marine" Lattimore is one of Southern California's premier fitness experts. A skilled personal trainer who privately trains professional athletes, celebrities, and community leaders, he has competed nationally as a bodybuilder. Tony's fitness expertise was featured in P90X and *The Daniel Plan in Action* fitness video series. His powerhouse workouts have a reputation for making fitness fun and exhilarating.

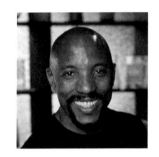

Kevin Forbes has a passion for inspiring others to build healthy habits and push through their physical and mental boundaries. Kevin has helped others grow as a personal trainer, group fitness instructor, and fitness professional. Most recently, he was a featured fitness instructor in *The Daniel Plan in Action* fitness video series. Kevin mentors not only future fitness leaders but also the foster youth in his local community.

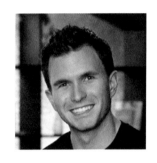

Janet Hertogh shares her love and enthusiasm for teaching in the classroom as an elementary school teacher and in a variety of fitness classes at Saddleback Church. Her passion for life change and transformation is a central theme wherever she goes. Her Masters Degree in Education along with her AFAA and personal training certification make her fully equipped to influence many. Janet was a featured fitness instructor in *The Daniel Plan in Action* fitness video series.

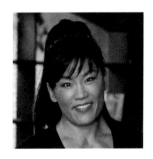

The Daniel Plan

40 Days to a Healthier Life

*Rick Warren D. Min., Daniel Amen M.D.,
Mark Hyman M.D.*

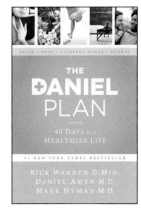

Revolutionize Your Health ... Once and for All.

During an afternoon of baptizing over 800 people, Pastor Rick Warren realized it was time for change. He told his congregation he needed to lose weight and asked if anyone wanted to join him. He thought maybe 200 people would sign up; instead he witnessed a movement unfold as 15,000 people lost over 260,000 pounds in the first year. With assistance from medical and fitness experts, Pastor Rick and thousands of people began a journey to transform their lives.

Welcome to The Daniel Plan.

Here's the secret sauce: The Daniel Plan is designed to be done in a supportive community relying on God's instruction for living.

When it comes to getting healthy, two are always better than one. Our research has revealed that people getting healthy together lose twice as much weight as those who do it alone. God never meant for you to go through life alone and that includes the journey to health.

Unlike the thousands of other books on the market, this book is not about a new diet, guilt-driven gym sessions, or shame-driven fasts. *The Daniel Plan* shows you how the powerful combination of faith, fitness, food, focus, and friends will change your health forever, transforming you in the most head-turning way imaginably — from the inside out.

Available in stores and online!

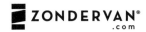

THE +DANIEL PLAN

The Daniel Plan Cookbook

Healthy Eating for Life

Rick Warren D. Min., Daniel Amen M.D., and Mark Hyman M.D. featuring The Daniel Plan Signature Chefs

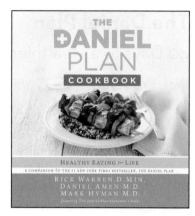

Based on *The Daniel Plan* book, *The Daniel Plan Cookbook: 40 Days to a Healthier Life* is a beautiful four-color cookbook filled with more than 100 delicious, Daniel Plan-approved recipes that offer an abundance of options to bring healthy cooking into your kitchen.

No boring drinks or bland entrées here. Get ready to enjoy appetizing, inviting, clean, simple meals to share in community with your friends and family.

Healthy cooking can be easy and delicious, and *The Daniel Plan Cookbook* is the mouth-watering companion to *The Daniel Plan* book and *The Daniel Plan Journal* to help transform your health in the most head-turning way imaginably — from the inside out.

Available in stores and online!

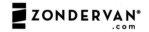

The Daniel Plan Journal

40 Days to a Healthier Life

Rick Warren and The Daniel Plan Team

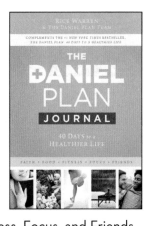

The Perfect Daniel Plan Companion for Better Overall Health

Research shows that tracking your food and exercise greatly contributes to your long-term success. Maximize your momentum by exploring and charting your journey through the five key Essentials of The Daniel Plan—Faith, Food, Fitness, Focus, and Friends.

Taking readers of *The Daniel Plan: 40 Days to a Healthier Life* to the next level, *The Daniel Plan Journal* is the perfect companion, providing encouraging reminders about your health. On the days you need a little boost, *The Daniel Plan Journal* has the daily Scripture, inspiration, and motivation you need to stay on track and keep moving forward.

Available in stores and online!

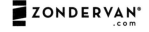

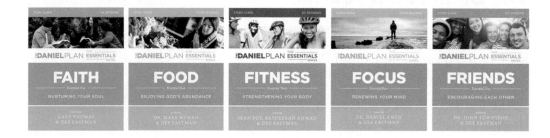

The Daniel Plan Five Essentials Series

The Daniel Plan Five Essentials Series is an innovative approach to creating a healthy lifestyle, rooted and framed by five life areas: Faith, Food, Fitness, Focus, and Friends.

Host Dee Eastman and The Daniel Plan's founding doctors and wellness faculty—including Gary Thomas, Dr. Mark Hyman, Sean Foy, Basheerah Ahmad, Dr. Daniel Amen, and Dr. John Townsend—equip you to make healthy choices on a daily basis.

Each video session features not only great teaching but testimony from those who have incorporated The Daniel Plan into their everyday lives. A weekly Fitness Move and Food Tip are also provided. The study guide include icebreakers and review questions, video notes, video discussion questions, next steps suggestions, prayer starters, and helpful appendices.

The Daniel Plan has transformed thousands of people around the world and it can transform you as well.

Available in stores and online!

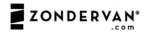

™DANIELPLAN

The Daniel Plan in Action
40 Day Fitness Programs With
Dynamic Workouts

Introduction by Rick Warren D. Min.

   The Daniel Plan in Action is a 40-day fitness
system with an innovative approach to creating a
healthy lifestyle, rooted and framed by five life areas:
faith, food, fitness, focus and friends. Three expert instructors
lead the variety of inspiring workouts with a strong backbone of faith and
community, complemented by a soundtrack of exclusive Christian music. This
4-session and 8-session systems focus on an abundance of healthy choices
offering you the encouragement and inspiration you need to succeed.

Go to DanielPlan.com now to learn more.

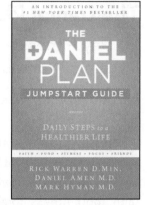

THE DANIEL PLAN

The Daniel Plan Jumpstart Guide

Daily Steps to a Healthier Life

Rick Warren D. Min., Daniel Amen M.D.,
Mark Hyman M.D.

The Daniel Plan Jumpstart Guide provides a bird's-eye view of getting your life on track to better health in five key areas: Faith, Food, Fitness, Focus, and Friends. This booklet provides all the key principles for readers to gain a vision for health and get started — breaking out existing content from *The Daniel Plan: 40 Days to a Healthier Life* into a 40-day action plan. The *Jumpstart Guide* encourages readers to use *The Daniel Plan* and *The Daniel Plan Journal* for more information and further success.

Available in stores and online!

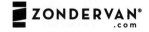